T0276986

Improve Your Health and Wellbeing

SUPER
QUICK
SKILLS

Improve Your Health and Wellbeing

Kaye
Rabel

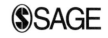

Los Angeles | London | New Delhi
Singapore | Washington DC | Melbourne

Los Angeles | London | New Delhi
Singapore | Washington DC | Melbourne

SAGE Publications Ltd
1 Oliver's Yard
55 City Road
London EC1Y 1SP

SAGE Publications Inc.
2455 Teller Road
Thousand Oaks, California 91320

SAGE Publications India Pvt Ltd
B 1/I 1 Mohan Cooperative Industrial Area
Mathura Road
New Delhi 110 044

SAGE Publications Asia-Pacific Pte Ltd
3 Church Street
#10-04 Samsung Hub
Singapore 049483

Editor: Jai Seaman
Assistant editor: Lauren Jacobs
Production editor: Rachel Burrows
Marketing manager: Catherine Slinn
Cover design: Shaun Mercier
Typeset by: C&M Digitals (P) Ltd, Chennai, India
Printed in the UK

Library of Congress Control Number: 2020942654

British Library Cataloguing in Publication data

A catalogue record for this book is available
from the British Library

ISBN 978-1-5297-4480-4

At SAGE we take sustainability seriously. Most of our products are printed in the UK using responsibly
sourced papers and boards. When we print overseas we ensure sustainable papers are used as measured
by the PREPS grading system. We undertake an annual audit to monitor our sustainability.

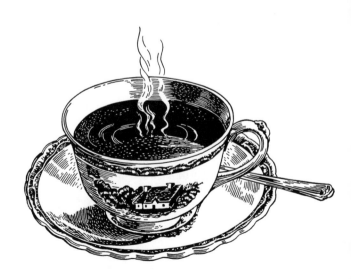

Contents

Everything in this book!

Section 4   How can I make sure I have a healthy mindset?

Having a healthy mindset plays a major part in successfully navigating difficult times and creating positive outcomes. This section details tools for improving and maintaining a healthy mindset.

Section 5   Why are healthy relationships important?

The relationships in our lives impact our overall health and wellbeing. This section discusses the significance of healthy relationships as well as the consequences of unhealthy relationships.

Section 6   How can I improve the relationships in my life?

Our relationships, like us, are not perfect. The relationships in our lives benefit us in many ways so it is important to make the best of them. This section provides tools for improving the relationships in your life.

Section 7   What does it mean to be connected to something more?

Connecting to more is a powerful way to find joy and personal fulfilment. This section discusses how to improve your wellbeing by recognising that it depends on more than just meeting your own individual needs.

Section 8   What are my personal goals for health and wellbeing?

Some people find it challenging to maintain improvements in their overall health. This section guides you through using goal setting as a tool to help you establish and maintain the improvements that you wish to make.

Section 9   What is alignment and how can I incorporate it into my life?

If you have ever been concerned about making sure you accomplish your goals in life, alignment is an essential component. This section discusses how our actions in different areas of our life align to achieve our health and wellness goals.

What is wellbeing?

10 second summary

Wellbeing refers to the overall health and wellness of an individual. The components that contribute to your wellbeing include both physical and mental wellbeing.

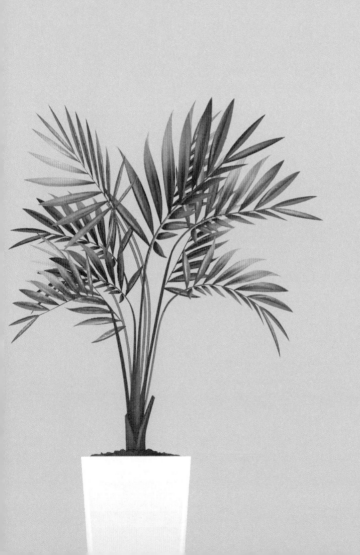

60 second summary

The components of health and wellness

Our physical wellbeing relates to the health of the body. Our diet or the food we eat and the amount of exercise we do impact the health of the body. The amount of rest we get also affects our physical health.

Our mental wellbeing includes our thoughts, relationships and a connection to something beyond ourselves. Our thoughts – in particular, the things we say to ourselves – affect our mental wellbeing. The people in our lives and the types of relationships we have also contribute to what we think about ourselves and affect our mind or mental wellbeing. Additionally, our purpose or desire to be connected to something beyond ourselves contributes to mental health too.

In this book you will learn tips and tools to help you look after your health and wellbeing now, while at university, and beyond.

What contributes to having a healthy body?

Proper nutrition and exercise contribute to having a healthy body. Nutrition can be defined as the nutrients you receive from consuming food. This includes vitamins, minerals, protein and fat. For optimal health and to feel your best, implement good nutritional habits and eat a healthy diet. A healthy diet includes eating vegetable, fruits and whole grains. If you consume animal proteins such as meat and dairy, it is suggested you select low fat options from this group. You will also need to limit processed food, foods and drinks high in sugar and foods high in fat. We will discuss more nutritional tips in Section 2.

It is also important to get an adequate amount of exercise. Exercise or physical activity includes cardiovascular exercise and resistance training. Cardiovascular exercise includes activities that elevate your heart rate beyond what it normally is when resting. Some examples of cardiovascular exercise include:

- Running or jogging
- Riding a bike or indoor cycling
- Swimming
- Football

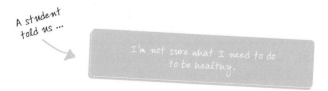

A student told us …

I'm not sure what I need to do to be healthy.

Resistance training includes activities such as lifting weights, using resistance bands or other types of training where the goal is to build muscle. In order to build muscle during resistance training, you lift weights or use some other form of resistance to fatigue your muscles. The body then works to repair the muscle and, as an adaptation, the muscle grows back stronger. We will talk more about this process as well as discuss more tips on how to exercise to improve your health in Section 3.

Rest is another component of your physical wellbeing. In our discussion in this book, we will also talk about rest in terms of alternating days of exercise with days of rest or less strenuous exercise.

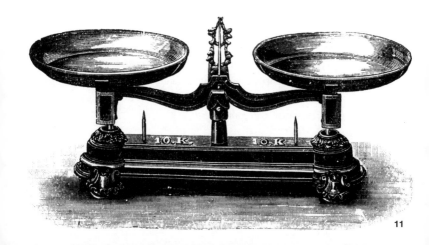

Having a healthy mind or mental wellbeing includes having healthy thoughts and relationships as well as being connected to something beyond ourselves. Please note that mental wellbeing can also be referred to as emotional wellbeing.

Thoughts in this context refers to what we say to ourselves. This includes the conversations we have in our heads about ourselves. For example, think about the last time you made a mistake. What did you say to yourself? Did you say something along the lines, of 'Wow, I can't believe I did that' or 'That was stupid'. We all have these sorts of conversations in our heads about ourselves and sometimes say negative things when we make a mistake or are unsure of how to do something. However, we must be careful to avoid overly negative thoughts or thinking only negative things. Constantly thinking in a negative way about yourself affects your mental wellbeing and mindset in an adverse way. This could possibly contribute to anxiety, low self-esteem and even depression. Although this pattern of thinking may have been a part of your life for some time, once you are aware of your thinking you have the capacity to incorporate more positive thoughts. Being aware of your thoughts helps you make positive changes.

The relationships we have in life also affect our wellbeing. Ultimately, the goal is to have relationships in your life that are positive and supportive. This includes relationships with your parents, siblings, other relatives, friends and a significant other. In Section 6, we will explore tips for optimizing the relationships in your life.

Finally, a *connection to more* refers to being connected to something larger than you as an individual. This can include:

- Soul/spirit – The concept of an individual being that goes beyond the physical body. Some may also believe that the soul is not bound by space or time.

- Higher power – A deity. This can also be described as a universal life force.

- Religion – The organized worship of a deity, deities or a higher power which usually includes the study of a sacred text and may also include rules and rituals.

- Charity – A nonprofit organization committed to promoting a social cause.

In Section 4, we will discuss tips and strategies for improving your mindset to improve your mental wellbeing.

Health isn't just about exercise and the food you eat, it's also the thoughts in your head!

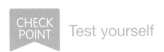

Test yourself

Test your knowledge by answering the following questions.

1 Wellbeing refers to the overall health and wellness of an individual. What are the components of wellbeing?

_____

_____

_____

2 What contributes to having a healthy body?

_____

_____

_____

3 What contributes to having a healthy mind?

_____

_____

_____

Answers

1. The components of wellbeing include physical and mental wellbeing. Physical wellbeing refers to the health of the body. Mental wellbeing includes our thoughts, relationships and a connection to something beyond ourselves.

2. Eating a healthy and nutrient rich diet, incorporating regular exercise and getting an adequate amount of rest contribute to maintaining a healthy body.

3. Having a healthy mind, or mental wellbeing, includes having healthy thoughts and relationships as well as being connected to something beyond ourselves.

How can I improve my health with nutrition?

10 second
summary

Your body uses nutrients for fuel as well as to repair the body. Determining if you have any nutritional deficits and eating a healthy diet can help you improve your health.

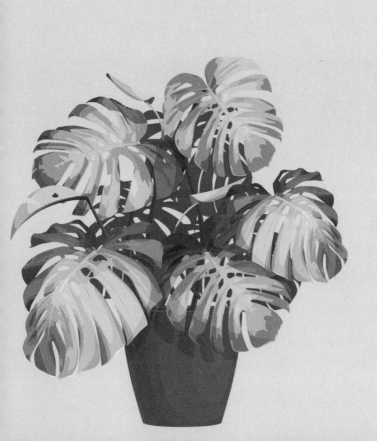

Food is fuel for your body

Nutrition plays a major role in our health. Food provides nutrients to your body so you can improve your health by changing your diet to incorporate more healthy food. This includes eating food primarily from wholefood, plant-based sources. You could have a blood test to check for any nutrient deficiencies and then supplement your diet to address any deficiencies. If we take a car as an example, it's like using the best petrol so your car runs at its best. Tips for improving your health with nutrition include:

- Incorporating as many wholefood, plant-based food sources as possible

- Limiting processed foods, meat, dairy, foods high in fat and foods high in sugar

- If possible, see a nutritionist to determine your specific micronutrient and caloric needs.

How does my body use food for nutrients?

Think of the human body as being like a car. In order for a car to run, the car needs fuel or an alternative power source. If it's poor quality, the car won't run well. The body carries out *metabolic functions*, meaning it takes the food we eat and converts it to fuel to keep it going. We need food for the organ systems in our body to work properly. Additionally, when we do other activities beyond resting, like running errands or going for a walk, our bodies need fuel from nutrients to support those activities. Think about what happens if you don't put fuel in your car or recharge it. The car will eventually stop and you won't be able to drive. In a similar way, when someone doesn't eat enough food they become malnourished and their body no longer functions properly. In the extreme instance of prolonged starvation, a person may even die. Food is an important part of maintaining your health.

A student told us ...

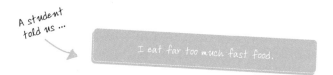

I eat far too much fast food.

In addition to supporting the metabolic functions that 'run' the body, the fuel that your body creates from the food you eat helps to repair the body.

 The cells that make up the tissues which in turn make up the organs in our bodies are constantly being repaired.

 The nutrients we take in from food support this process.

 Eating healthy food helps to provide an optimal level of nutrients to your body so it can work at its best.

What does 'wholefood, plant-based' mean?

Wholefood refers to the original unprocessed or minimally processed plant. For example, if you buy an apple, the apple is a wholefood. But if you buy a frozen apple pie, you are buying processed food. Plant-based foods include vegetables, fruits, wholegrains, beans, legumes and nuts. Eating a wholefood, plant-based diet is considered healthy because it avoids processed food, which can be high in fat, sodium and sugar. Wholefood, plant-based diets also provide nutrients rich in vitamins and minerals. In addition to minimizing the amount of processed food you eat, it is a good idea to limit meat, dairy, foods high in fat and foods high in sugar. It doesn't mean you can't eat these things at all, but you do want to restrict your intake.

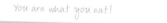

You are what you eat!

How do I find out my micronutrient and calorific needs?

It may be helpful to arrange a blood test to look at your overall health including how your organs are functioning and if you have any nutrient deficiencies. A nutrient deficiency is when you are not getting enough of the recommended amount of a particular vitamin or mineral. If it is determined that you are deficient in a particular micronutrient (vitamins and minerals) there may be supplements that you can take. A dietitian or nutritionist can advise you about what foods to eat or vitamins or minerals to take.

It is important to be attuned to how your body responds to different foods, as well as any changes in your overall wellbeing. Many people may have a gluten or diary intolerance for instance, or a vitamin or nutrient deficiency, and not realise it. If you feel a change in how your body responds to a particular food at any point, or if you feel noticeably different but can't identify why, go to your GP who will be able to provide some assistance in identifying whether any intolerances or deficiencies are present.

Dietitians and nutritionists can provide guidance on your specific calorific needs. If you don't eat enough calories your body won't function properly. If you eat too many calories, your body will store these calories as fat and you may gain weight. So, taking in the right number of calories is important as well. The number of calories you eat is based on what's called your metabolic rate – or how many calories your body burns in a day while carrying out metabolic functions. A nutritionist can also help you modify your caloric intake if your goal is to lose or gain weight. For example, in order to lose weight, you will need to create a calorific deficit. You can create a deficit in calories by combining a reduction of the calories you eat with exercise. A nutritionist can help you determine your metabolic rate and your optimal calorie intake in order to safely lose or gain weight, if this is advised.

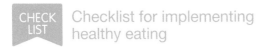

CHECK LIST Checklist for implementing healthy eating

☐ Eat wholefood, plant-based food sources

☐ Limit processed foods, meat, dairy, foods high in fat and foods high in sugar

☐ If possible, see a nutritionist to determine your specific micronutrient and calorific needs

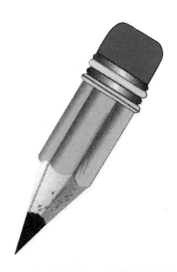

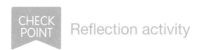

CHECK POINT Reflection activity

What are some things you can change about your diet in order to eat more healthily? Review the following and detail your responses in the space provided below.

Thinking about your current diet …

1   What components of your diet would you consider healthy?

_____

_____

_____

2   What might be unhealthy?

_____

_____

_____

3   How can you modify your diet in order to eat more healthily?

_____

_____

_____

Congratulations

on learning tools for improving your nutrition!

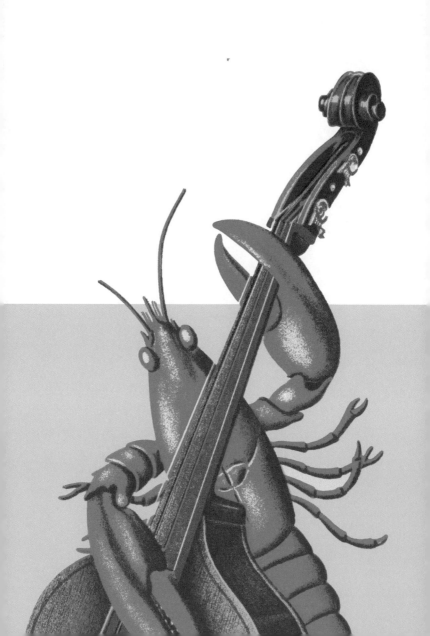

How can I improve my health with a balance of exercise and rest?

10 second summary

The organs and systems that make up our bodies benefit from regular exercise. For optimal health, you should incorporate regular exercise but also ensure you get enough rest.

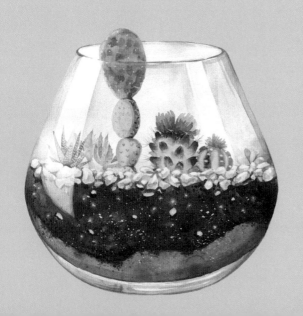

60 second
summary

Balance is the key

The human body was made to move. Incorporating regular exercise into your lifestyle can improve your health. Your heart, muscles and bones benefit from regular physical activity. As we previously discussed, physical activity includes both cardiovascular exercise and resistance training.

As the name suggests, cardiovascular exercise helps improve the overall health of the cardiovascular system, which includes the heart. Resistance exercise or training helps to improve the musculoskeletal system which includes muscles and bones.

However, like most things, exercise should not be overdone. It is important to incorporate rest days in your exercise regimen. Rest days, in this context, means adding in days when you purposefully don't exercise. This gives your body time to recover. We will talk more about this process later in this section.

The goal of cardiovascular exercise is to elevate your heart rate above your resting heart rate for a sustained period of time. Your resting heart rate is the number of times your heart beats per minute. Factors including your age and level of cardiovascular fitness will influence this number. Runners or other athletes who frequently train their cardiovascular systems will have a lower resting heart rate – for example, their resting heart rate may be around 40 beats per minute. Someone who doesn't exercise and generally has a sedentary lifestyle will have a higher resting heart rate. This person's resting heart rate could potentially be around 90–100 beats per minute. In this case it is more than double than that of someone who does regular cardiovascular exercise and means that this person's heart must work harder when they do exercise.

When you exercise, you heart rate will fluctuate between what's called aerobic and anaerobic exercise. *Aerobic* means in the presence of oxygen, where you are breathing and able to hold a conversation with at least short responses. When doing aerobic cardiovascular exercise you should do it for at least 30 minutes. You can do aerobic cardiovascular exercise daily, or at least 3–4 times per week. Common exercises include:

- Jogging/running

- Brisk/speed walking

- Cycling or riding a stationary bike

- Using an elliptical

- Rowing.

Anaerobic means without oxygen, where someone is putting in maximum effort. This person would generally be working so hard they would not be able to speak. This happens during activities such as sprinting or running quickly up a flight of stairs. You can only do these types of exercises for a short period of time. You will also feel out of breath when you stop.

There is a type of cardiovascular training that incorporates both aerobic and anaerobic activity called high-intensity interval training or HIIT. The benefits of HIIT include burning fat in shorter training sessions. These workouts should not be done for longer than 20 minutes including warm-up and cool-down. A HIIT workout alternates between anaerobic and aerobic exercise. An example of a HIIT workout would be alternating between sprinting for 20 seconds and jogging or walking for 40 seconds. Walking or jogging gives you a break to bring your heart rate back down and gets you ready for the next interval. Do intervals consecutively. An example of an HITT workout is:

- Warm-up: 3-minute jog

- Interval (repeat 10 times): sprint for 20 seconds, walk for 40 seconds

- Cool-down: 2-minute walk.

Be sure to stretch following workouts to prevent excessive soreness!

It is also a good idea to buy and use a heart-rate monitor during physical activity to track your heart rate and chart your progress. Be sure to also consult your doctor before starting an exercise programme to ensure you don't have any conditions that could be adversely affected by exercise.

CHECK LIST Checklist for cardiovascular exercise

☐ Consult your doctor before starting a new exercise programme

☐ Do aerobic cardiovascular exercise at least 3 times a week for at least 30 minutes each time

☐ Keep high-intensity interval training (HIIT) under 20 minutes

☐ Be sure to cool down after workouts and to stretch

☐ Use a heart-rate monitor to chart your progress

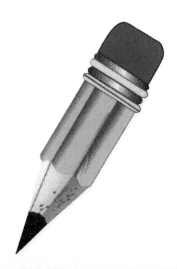

How can I incorporate resistance training and rest?

The goal of resistance training is to strengthen and build muscle. During resistance training you do repetitions using weights or resistance bands. This stresses the muscles and causes microtrauma in them. Your body responds to this microtrauma by repairing the muscles and making them stronger in order to adapt to the training. This is how we build muscle. It is also why you need to incorporate rest into your resistance training regimen! For example, if you do a weightlifting workout that targets your chest and triceps on Monday, you shouldn't work those same muscles on Tuesday. To give your body time to repair your muscles and flush out the lactic acid that builds up as a result of resistance training, it is a good idea to lift weights every other day.

In resistance training, form and proper technique are very important in order to maximize your weightlifting effort and prevent injury. Always be sure to warm-up properly prior to a workout and stretch afterwards. To help you make the most of resistance training and to make sure you are working out safely it may be helpful to seek out the help of a qualified personal trainer to provide guidance on proper weightlifting techniques. This may of course be an expensive option so please do ensure that you have the means to do this.

Exercise is an investment in the priceless asset that is your health!

Checklist for resistance training

☐ To get started with resistance training, consider seeking out the help of a qualified personal trainer

☐ Warm up prior to training

☐ Be sure to use proper form and technique to prevent injuries

☐ Be sure to rest and not train the same muscle group on consecutive days

☐ Stretch following your workout

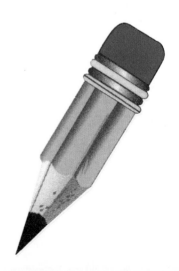

What are some additional resources?

Visit the NHS website at www.nhs.uk for more information and tools to help you improve your health and wellbeing. In addition to resources for overall health and ways to eat a healthy diet, the NHS provides resources for both cardiovascular and resistance training. You can also find a free library of exercises at www.acefitness.org/education-and-resources/life style/exercise-library

A student told us ...

I have more energy when I exercise.

CHECK POINT Cardiovascular exercise and resistance training

1   **True or False**   Anaerobic exercise can be sustained for longer durations than aerobic exercise.

2   **True or False**   Your resting heart rate will decrease as your cardiovascular fitness improves.

3   **True or False**   Because the quadriceps is a large muscle, it's okay to train it on Thursday and then again the next day on Friday.

4   **True or False**   You should ensure that you are using proper form and technique.

Answers:
1 False
2 True
3 False
4 True

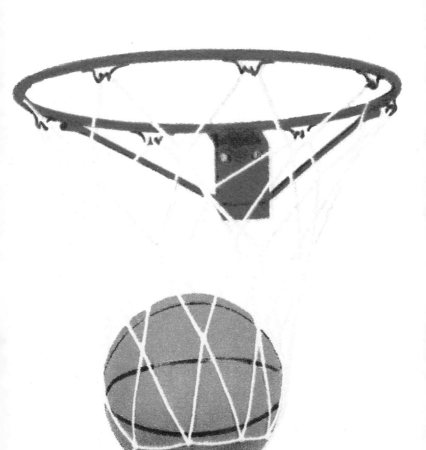

How can I make sure I have a healthy mindset?

10 second summary

Having a healthy mindset includes:

- Seeing yourself in a positive way
- Using strategies to help you have empowering thoughts
- Responding instead of reacting to challenging situations that occur in life.

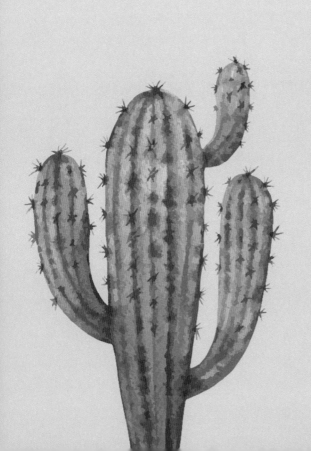

The mindset of responding versus reacting

Mindset is the way your think about life, how you view situations and your overall outlook on life. It includes your underlying values and how you relate to life as it happens to you.

Having a healthy mindset means seeing yourself in a positive way where you are in control of your life and the things that happen to you. With a healthy mindset, you have thoughts that help you respond to life's challenges in empowering ways. This includes responding versus reacting. When you *respond* to a challenging situation you evaluate the situation and determine the best actions based on benefits as well as the related consequences or costs. When you *react* you have a spur-of-the-moment reaction to a difficult situation without thinking about the consequences. It isn't always easy to respond versus react in the moment of a difficult or challenging situation in life, but having a healthy mindset helps you make the right choice when it matters the most.

You may be thinking what about things that happen in our lives that are beyond our control, like the COVID-19 pandemic or natural disasters such as the 2020 forest fires in Australia. When it comes to these kinds of situations, mindset refers to how you respond. With a healthy mindset, although you may be concerned and stressed, you find ways to address challenges in empowering ways.

For instance, during the COVID-19 pandemic with mandatory quarantines people faced a lot of uncertainty about how long the lockdown would last and how they would spend their time. Someone with a less healthy mindset may get depressed, withdraw, and maybe even adopt unhealthy coping mechanisms such as excessive drinking or substance abuse. Someone with a healthy mindset, although just as stressed as the person in the previous example, would find constructive ways to use their time like learning a new language, researching and doing home workouts on YouTube, or learning how to cook. Challenging situations are a part of life, and having a healthy mindset is very helpful in navigating difficult times.

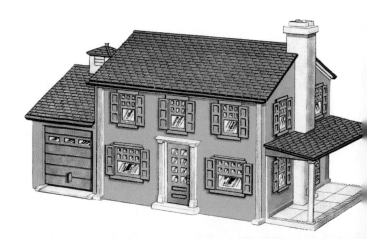

What's the difference between healthy, empowering thoughts and negative thoughts?

Your thoughts create your mindset. We all have negative thoughts and must learn how to address those thoughts and replace them with healthier ones. Healthy, empowering thoughts are centred around creative outcomes. Healthy thoughts are positive. They give life to new possibilities or perspectives. Examples of healthy, empowering thoughts include:

- I can do this.

- This is challenging but I will work it out.

- Things may not look the best, but they will get better.

- I trust myself.

- I believe in myself.

- I love myself.

Negative thoughts are the opposite of healthy, empowering thoughts. They do not seek to create positive outcomes and only dwell on the negative aspects of a situation. Negative thoughts inhibit you from being your best and creating positive outcomes. Examples of negatives thoughts include:

- I am not good at anything.

- I'm going to fail so I might as well not even try.

- This is too hard.

Having a healthy mindset helps you truly to be the best version of yourself and achieve the things you want in life. So now let's look at how to overcome negative thinking.

Everyone has negative thoughts but people with healthy mindsets have learned how to replace those negative thoughts with healthy thoughts. In order to overcome negative thinking, you must first learn how to become aware that you are having these thoughts. By being self-aware and observing your thoughts you can reflect on the types of thoughts you are having. Becoming self-aware, observing and reflecting on your thinking is a process that takes time and patience to learn. However, once you learn the process and how to overcome negative thinking, you will be able to make meaningful improvements to your mindset. Activities such as journaling will help you observe and reflect on your thinking. During journaling, you can also work on overcoming negative thoughts by identifying and replacing them with positive thoughts. Let's take a closer look at journaling as well as some other techniques.

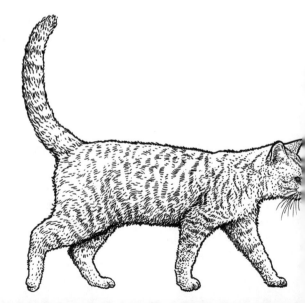

Journaling

Journaling is a technique that will help you learn how to replace negative thoughts in a structured way.

- **Write the negative thought.** Write down the negative thought on which you've been ruminating.

- **Write the source.** Next, try to think about the source of that thought.

- **Write a reassuring thought.** Reassure yourself that things will be okay.

- **Write a replacement empowering thought.** Think about ways you can create a new empowering thought to replace the negative thought.

- **Write what you will do next.** Lastly, think of and list what you can do next to make the empowering thought come to life.

An example journal entry may look like this:

- **Negative thought:** I am so overwhelmed, I don't know how I'm going to get all of this done.

- **Source:** I feel overwhelmed because I have a lot of things to do and I am not sure what to do first.

- **Reassurance:** Okay, it's going to be okay. There is a solution.

- **Empowering thought:** I can do this. I can get through this.

- **What can I do next?** I can create a to-do list and do one thing at a time until I have completed everything. That will help me focus on getting things done and alleviate stress.

Other ways to overcome negative thinking include:

- Sticky note reminders

- Practising gratitude

- Practising calmness

- Speaking with a therapist or counsellor.

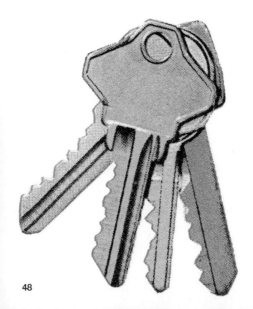

Sticky note reminder

Writing a positive thought on a sticky note helps you quickly replace a negative thought. Whenever you continue to have a negative thought, think of an empowering thought to replace it. Write the empowering thought on a sticky note and place it somewhere you'll see it often. Look at the sticky note whenever that particular negative thought comes into your mind. Soon you will start to automatically think of the positive thought without looking at the sticky note!

Practise gratitude

Practising gratitude also helps with having a healthier mindset. Start each day by spending time reflecting on what you are thankful for in your life. In the morning when you wake up think of 3–7 things you are grateful for and say them out loud. When you focus on what is good, it is typically difficult to focus on the negative at the same time.

Healthy thoughts give life to positive outcomes.

Practise calmness

Practising calmness and making time for quiet moments contribute to a healthy mindset as well. The calmness practice will also help calm the mind and enable you to respond rather than react in difficult situations. Some techniques to practise calmness include:

- Meditating

- Listening to music

- Aromatherapy.

Speak with a therapist

Lastly but importantly, you are also advised to speak to a professional therapist or counsellor to learn additional strategies for having a healthy mindset. You can also visit Mind at www.mind.org.uk for information on mental wellbeing.

A student told us ...

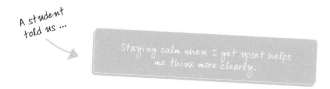

Staying calm when I get upset helps me think more clearly.

CHECK LIST Checklist for maintaining a healthy mindset

☐ Eat a healthy diet

☐ Exercise

☐ Focus on responding vs reacting

☐ Journal

☐ Practise gratitude

☐ Practise calmness

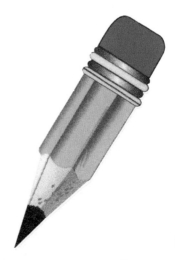

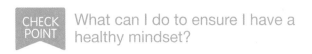

CHECK POINT What can I do to ensure I have a healthy mindset?

Using the space provided below, detail how you can ensure you have a healthy mindset.

_____

_____

_____

_____

_____

_____

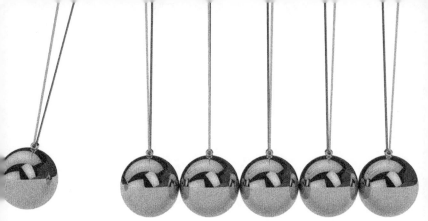

Why are healthy relationships important?

10 second summary

Healthy relationships provide love, support and companionship. Humans are social creatures and healthy relationships help fulfil our social needs in a positive way.

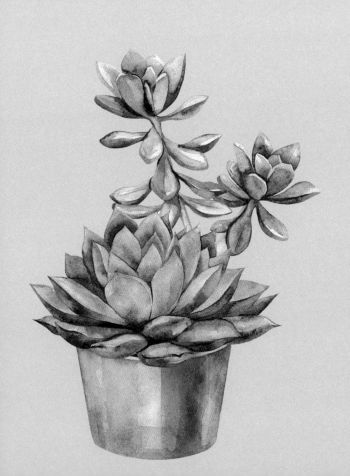

Healthy relationships provide companionship and support

Human beings are highly social creatures and having a sense of belonging is essential for our overall wellbeing. Healthy relationships facilitate this sense of belonging by providing companionship and support. In healthy relationships, people are genuinely concerned for one another. Healthy relationships also provide love and encouragement.

Companionship comprises having conversations and spending time with someone. During this time, you should do things that both people enjoy. Companionship also includes support, help and reliability.

What are the benefits of conversations?

Conversations provide an opportunity for emotional bonding by learning more about the other person and understanding their emotions and feelings. Through conversations we help each other grow as well as feel heard.

Conversations include:

- Discussions about what is happening in each other's lives

- Opportunities to express ourselves and listen to others

- Opportunities to contribute when the listener shares their ideas and insights about what's going on in our lives.

What does it mean to feel supported?

Feeling supported means being able to rely on someone to be there when you need them. This support can include:

- Help when needed

- Encouragement through words and actions

- A source of love and compassion.

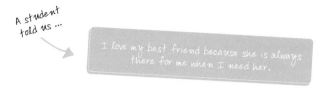
What are the components of healthy relationships?

Platonic relationships are solely based on friendship whereas romantic relationships go beyond a friendship to include physical attraction and/or a sexual relationship. Regardless of whether a relationship is platonic or romantic, healthy relationships contain the following components:

- Genuine interest in your life and wellbeing

- Reciprocity

- Love, support and encouragement

- Open lines of communication

- Reliability, trust and security.

Genuine interest in your life and wellbeing

Having a genuine interest in your life and wellbeing means having a real concern for your life and the things that are happening in it. It means being excited for you when good things happen and showing empathy when you are going through difficult times.

Reciprocity

Reciprocity means there is a healthy give-and-take in the relationship. Both people benefit from the relationship. For example, both people listen to each other. The relationship isn't one-sided where person A always listens but when person A wants to talk, person B is always busy. Both people are there for each other.

Love, support and encouragement

Love involves truly caring for a person – their health and wellbeing is important to you. With love, you seek to treat the other person as you wish to be treated. Love includes respect for each other as an individual as well as respect for each other's boundaries. As a part of love no one feels forced into things or manipulated into doing something they don't want to do.

People in healthy relationships support and encourage one another with words and actions. This includes providing words of encouragement when either of you is having a bad day or going through a difficult time. It also includes doing nice things for each other without wanting something in return.

Open lines of communication

In healthy relationships, the lines of communication are open. You should feel comfortable sharing your feelings without the other person ridiculing you, becoming angry or not listening. People can openly share and listen to each other in a productive way when both feel that they are heard and that their feelings matter.

Reliability, trust and security

In healthy relationships people can rely on each other. People don't disappear or ghost each other for periods of time. These kinds of behaviours are the opposite of being reliable and are not healthy. Reliability also includes following through and keeping your word. If someone consistently breaks promises it becomes difficult to develop trust in a relationship. In a healthy relationship you feel secure. If you don't trust the other person, it is not possible to have any sense of security. As a part of feeling secure you should feel safe in the relationship both mentally and physically. We will talk more about steps to improve relationships in the next section. However, it is important not to remain in any relationship where you fear for your personal safety.

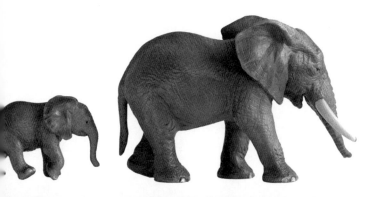

What are the consequences of unhealthy relationships?

Unhealthy relationships can turn into what are called *toxic relationships*. These kinds of relationships have been termed toxic because they damage your overall wellbeing instead of helping it. These relationships are generally the opposite of healthy relationships. If you are in a relationship that lacks any of the following, you may not be in a healthy relationship:

- Genuine interest in your life and wellbeing

- Reciprocity

- Love, support and encouragement

- Open lines of communication

- Reliability, trust and security.

A relationship lacking these components can cause stress and adversely affect your health and mental wellbeing. We will discuss how to address these kinds of relationships in Section 6.

The people in your life should build you up not bring you down.

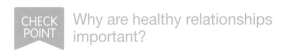

Why are healthy relationships important?

Let's check your understanding of it all. Test your knowledge by answering the following questions.

1   Why are healthy relationships important?

    a   They are the sole means of having high self-esteem

    b   They are a source of love, support and companionship

    c   They provide a source of financial support

2   Relationships provide companionship by allowing you to:

    a   Engage in conversations that facilitate emotional bonding

    b   Spend time with someone only because you feel lonely

    c   Consistently break promises because the other person is very understanding

3   Which of the following is *not* a component of a healthy relationship?

    a   Supporting and encouraging one another with words and actions

    b   Respecting each other's personal boundaries

    c   Not sharing your feelings out of fear the other person will get upset

4   What are some potential consequences of unhealthy relationships?

    a   Harm to your wellbeing

    b   No real consequences

    c   Increase in your communication skills

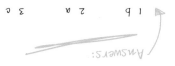

Answers: 1 b   2 a   3 c   4 a

How can I improve the relationships in my life?

10 second summary

Improving relationships in your life starts with evaluating the health of a relationship to determine if it works for your life. Next you can implement communication strategies to help improve the relationships you want to have.

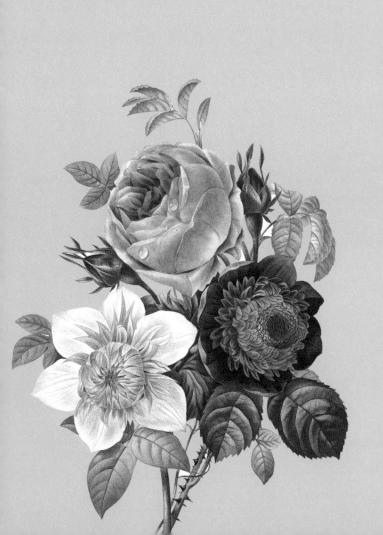

60 second summary

How to improve relationships

The first step to improving the relationships in your life is to first evaluate the overall health of a relationship. You may find that you need to end some of the relationships in your life, while others can be worked on.

If a relationship includes most of the components of a healthy relationship that you read about in Section 5 (see p. 59), you can implement communication strategies to help optimize the relationship. In order to improve relationships, both people must value the relationship, be open to honest communication and active listening, and be committed to following through and doing their part to make things better.

Value the relationship enough to work on it

In order to improve the relationship, both parties must value and see the benefits of the relationship. Both people need to want to have the other person in their life as well as have a genuine interest in making the relationship work. This provides the motivation that is required to work on the relationship.

Both people in the relationship must be willing to do the following:

- Value the relationship enough to work on it.

- Be open to honest communication.

- Be open to active listening.

- Be committed to improving the relationship and following through.

Honest and open communication is key. Both people must have a desire to put in the work to improve the relationship.

Honest communication

It is also important that both people honestly and openly share what they need from the relationship or what they would like to see change. Therefore, both parties need to work to create a non-judgmental environment for sharing. As a suggestion, it may be helpful for both people to write down their thoughts prior to speaking and then take turns sharing.

Actively listen to each other

A major component of the improvement process is actively listening to each other. Active listening means devoting your full attention to what the recipient is saying, making an effort to hear out the other person, and trying to understand their perspective. During active listening it is important to paraphrase what the other person said to confirm you interpreted what was shared as the other person intended. It is important not to become defensive or judgmental and to hear the other person's perspective. It is also a good idea to ensure you have a positive mindset and focus on responding versus reacting in order to listen effectively.

Be committed to improving the relationship and following through

After sharing and agreeing on what is needed to improve the relationship each person must be committed to doing their part. Both people need to follow through in order for this process to be effective.

> Relationships work best when people are committed to working on them.

CHECK LIST   Checklist for improving both platonic and romantic relationships

- [ ] Be open to honest communication

- [ ] Be open to active listening

- [ ] Agree on what is needed from both people to improve the relationship

- [ ] Try to see things from the other person's perspective

- [ ] Be committed to improving the relationship and following through

- [ ] Focus on responding versus reacting

- [ ] Set personal boundaries if needed

Now, let's reflect on how you can work on a relationship in your life.

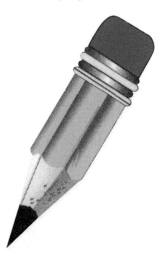

What if a relationship is toxic or unhealthy?

Unfortunately, there are times in life when you will need to end a relationship because it does not contribute to your wellbeing. In Section 5 (see p. 62) we learnt that if your relationship lacks any of the following it may not be a healthy relationship:

- Genuine interest in your life and wellbeing

- Reciprocity

- Love, support and encouragement

- Open lines of communication

- Reliability, trust and security.

It is not advisable to remain in a relationship in which people make you feel bad or uncomfortable. You should also not remain in a relationship where you do not feel safe. It can be helpful to speak to a qualified professional such as a therapist or counsellor to work on ways to exit an unsafe relationship. You should also discuss and explore the healing process for any emotional trauma you may have suffered.

There may be relationships with family members where completely removing the person from your life is difficult. Again, discuss the situation with a therapist or counsellor and work on ways to establish boundaries and limit interactions.

A student told us ...

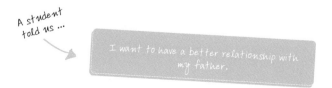

I want to have a better relationship with my father.

CHECK POINT How can you improve a relationship?

1   Think about the relationships in your life and select at least one: _____

2   Review the components of healthy relationships:

   a   Genuine interest in your life and wellbeing

   b   Reciprocity

   c   Love, support and encouragement

   d   Open lines of communication

   e   Reliability, trust and security.

3   Which components might benefit from improvements in this relationship:

_____

_____

_____

4   Action plan:

   a   Review the strategies discussed in this section for improving relationships.

   b   Select at least two strategies and discuss how you will use the strategy to improve the relationship(s) you selected.

Strategy 1: _____

I will use it by:

_____

_____

_____

Strategy 2: _____

I will use it by:

_____

_____

_____

Strategy 3: _____

I will use it by:

_____

_____

_____

Congratulations

on developing strategies to improve your relationships!

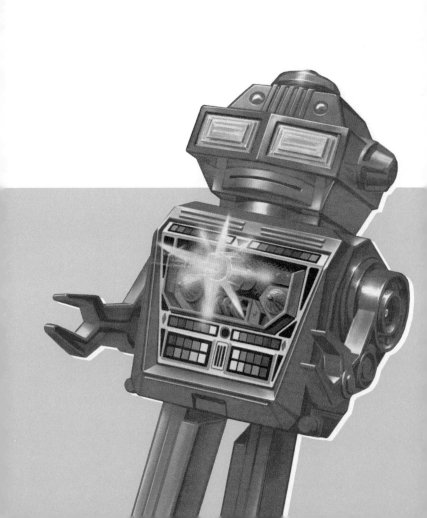

What does it mean to be connected to something more?

10 second summary

A connection to more is the recognition that life goes beyond meeting your own individual needs. The core values that guide your life will typically be associated with this connection.

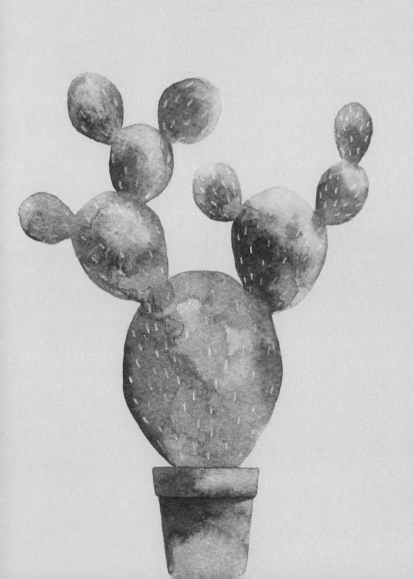

Being connected to more

Being connected to more relates to having a connection that goes beyond your life at the individual level. It is the recognition that life goes beyond meeting your own individual needs. This may include recognizing and feeling a sense of connection to a higher power. A higher power may include a deity or deities. It may also include being in touch with the concept of your soul and an association with the universe.

Being connected to more can also include the desire to make a difference in your community, the world or a particular social cause. There is typically a relationship between this connection to more and your core values and belief system.

What are core my values?

Core values refer to the principles and beliefs that guide your life. These may be derived from a more formal belief system such as an organized religion or from a sacred text. You may have adopted these core values from your parents or discovered them on your own.

Examples of core values include:

- Treating other people as you wish to be treated

- Showing kindness and compassion to others

- Always doing the right thing even when no one is watching

- Having balance in life

- Family being important

- Having a belief in a higher power or deity.

A student told us ...

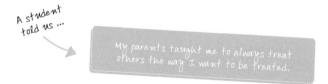

My parents taught me to always treat others the way I want to be treated.

Why is it important to be connected to more?

Having a connection to something more is important because this relationship provides a sense of purpose. Having a sense of purpose in life contributes to your wellbeing as a human because it provides a way for you to contribute to something beyond your individual experience.

Some additional benefits of this connection include making friends and establishing relationships with others who also have a similar purpose. These connections with people enrich and help make life's journey more fulfilling. If you only live at the individual level it may be difficult to relate to your community or the larger world. It may be difficult to have an understanding of your purpose in life. As part of being connected to more, particularly with contributing to your community or causes, it feels good to devote your time and resources. Although you are helping to further the efforts of an organization or cause, you may find it very personally fulfilling to be involved in these activities.

Extraordinary things can also result from being connected to more. Think about individuals such as Mahatma Gandhi, Mother Teresa or Martin Luther King Jr. They devoted their lives to fulfilling their purpose which was associated with something beyond their individual lives. All three became very prominent figures in history because they helped transform the lives of people around the world, illustrating that great things can result when we work to fulfil our purpose in life.

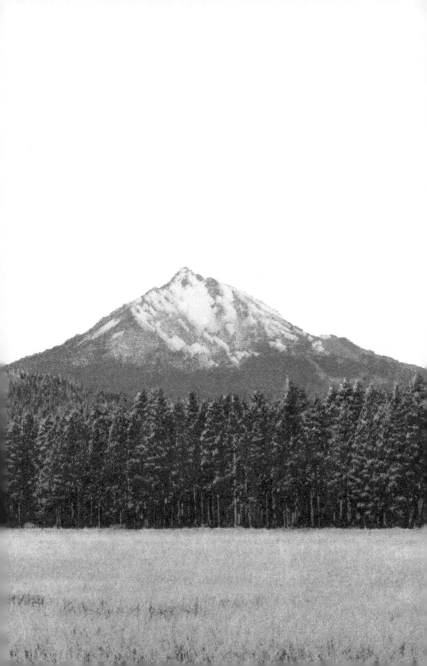

What is my purpose?

Your purpose in life can be derived from how you see your life helping others. You may have a particular talent or skill that you can use to help others. For example:

A musician

Carlos loves to write and play music. People have shared with Carlos that his music makes them happy. Carlos says his purpose is to make people happier through his music.

A personal trainer

Sara is a personal trainer. She helps people live healthier lifestyles. Sara feels her purpose in life is to help people be healthier.

Now, let's reflect on your core values and purpose.

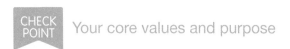
CHECK POINT Your core values and purpose

Take some time to think how you are connected to more.

Using the space below, list three connections and discuss why they are important to you.

1   Connection: _____

Why is it important?

_____

_____

_____

2   Connection: _____

Why is it important?

_____

_____

_____

3   Connection: _____

Why is it important?

_____

_____

_____

Take some time to think about what you are good at and enjoy doing.

1   How can these things help others?

_____

_____

_____

2   What could potentially be your purpose?

_____

_____

_____

3   Detail some things that could potentially be your purpose. Please
    note that this may not be very clear and may take time for you to
    clarify! Right now, what is important is thinking about your purpose
    and brainstorming ideas. Over time you will be able to clarify your
    purpose more clearly.

_____

_____

_____

What are my personal health and wellbeing goals?

10 second summary

There will be times in life when you need to make improvements to your health and wellbeing. Setting goals is a great way to monitor and track your progress.

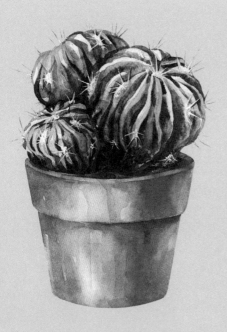

60 second summary

Health and wellbeing goals

As we get older and go through different experiences in our lives, our health and wellbeing needs change. It is important to periodically evaluate your health and wellbeing.

In instances where you need to make improvements in either area or both, goal setting is a useful tool. Setting goals is helpful for not only improving your health and wellbeing but also maintaining it. Examples of goals include:

Health

- Exercise at least 4 times a week in order to improve my physical health.

- Work with a nutritionist to improve my diet to lower my cholesterol level by 10 points by next year.

Wellbeing

- Practise gratitude by reflecting on 7 things I am grateful for each morning.

- Write a daily journal entry and replace a negative thought with a positive thought.

How do I set goals for my health and wellbeing?

In order to set health and wellbeing goals, you must first assess where you are.

You can have annual check-ups to evaluate your health. From a wellbeing perspective, you can monitor and reflect on how you are feeling. This gives insight into your overall wellness.

Next, you will need to determine:

1   What improvements you want to make (you will need to be specific about what it is that you want to change)

2   The timeframe in which you would like to see the improvement

3   How you will do it.

Ultimately, you need to be able to track your progress and determine when you have achieved your goal. It may take months or possibly a year to achieve a goal.

There are some goals you will be able to complete daily, such as the example above of writing a daily journal entry. In that instance, you would complete the goal daily and it would be something you do every day to maintain your mindset. You will never stop having negative thoughts – they are just a part of life – but when you are more aware of them and practise replacing negative thoughts with positive ones you work on your mindset. In this sense, the work is ongoing practice.

> Goals are like a map ... they help get you to where you want to go.

Tips for setting goals include

- Identify an area of improvement – a specific statement of what you would like to improve.

- Consider the time frame – a specific statement of when goal will be achieved.

- Itemise actions – a specific statement of what you will do to facilitate the improvement.

A student told us ...

> I like setting goals because it gives me something to work towards.

1   Review the goals below and identify the following for each goal:

-   Area of improvement

-   Possible time frame

-   Actions to create the change.

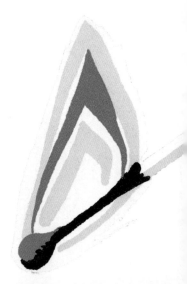

Goal: Exercise at least 4 times a week in order to improve my physical health		
Area of improvement	**Time frame**	**Actions**

Goal: Work with a nutritionist to improve my diet to reduce my cholesterol by 10 points by next year		
Area of improvement	**Time frame**	**Actions**

Goal: Practise gratitude by reflecting on 7 things I am grateful for every morning		
Area of improvement	**Time frame**	**Actions**

Goal: Write a daily journal entry and replace a negative thought with a positive thought		
Area of improvement	**Time frame**	**Actions**

Now, let's reflect on your goals.

2   What are your health and wellbeing goals?

- Take some time to think about your health and wellbeing.

- In what areas would you like to make some improvements?

- What goals can you set to make these improvements?

- Using the space below, detail 3 personal goals. Be sure to include:

  a   Area of improvement

  b   Possible time frame

  c   Actions to create the change.

Goal 1: _____

_____

_____

_____

Goal 2: _____

_____

_____

_____

Goal 3: _____

_____

_____

_____

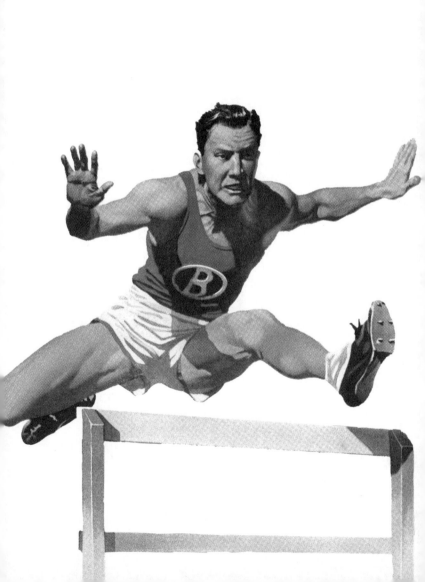

What is alignment and how can I incorporate it into my life?

10 second summary

Alignment includes making sure you are taking the right actions to accomplish your goals. A lack of alignment jeopardizes effectively achieving your goals.

60 second
summary

The definition of alignment

Alignment relates to ensuring that all the actions that you undertake are consistent with achieving a bigger task or goal. So, making sure all the components of your health and wellbeing align means examining your health goals as well as your wellbeing goals and making sure they are consistent with each other.

For instance, it is not in alignment if you say you want to improve your overall health but have no plans to address your nutrition when you have some unhealthy eating habits. Think of alignment in terms of a machine working at optimal performance. All of the components work together to help you be your best self.

Alignment plays an important part in achieving goals. There will be times in life when you need to make improvements to your health and well-being. Setting goals helps you monitor and track your progress. Being conscious of and ensuring what you do aligns with your intentions helps you to achieve your goals.

When you set out to accomplish a goal, there are subtasks or actions that add up to attaining the overall goal. If these tasks are not consistent with the accomplishment of the goal, you may find that it takes longer than you anticipated to achieve the goal. Unfortunately, there can even be instances of so much misalignment that you never achieve the goal. We set goals because we have a desire to achieve them.

With alignment, your actions are consistent with your intentions. Mis-alignment happens when our actions are inconsistent with our intentions for accomplishing a task or goal. Let's review some examples of align-ment and misalignment.

> Alignment means having a clear path to attaining your goals!

Examples of alignment

- Studying to prepare for an exam is in alignment with doing well on the test.

- Including exercise as a part of your weekly routine is in alignment with living a healthy lifestyle.

Examples of misalignment

- Having coffee before you go to bed is not in alignment with falling asleep easily.

- Eating unlimited processed food is not in alignment with living a healthy lifestyle.

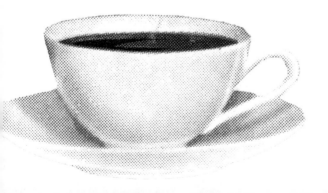

In the previous section, we examined goal setting and discussed the components of goals. One of those components was the actions that you undertake to achieve the goal. The goal statement included the main action for achieving the goal, but it didn't include every little single thing that you need do or not do. We can call these *sub-actions*. For example, in the following goal the ultimate goal is to improve your physical wellbeing:

> Exercise at least 4 times a week in order to improve my physical health.

The action to accomplish this goal is to exercise at least 4 times per week. While exercising is the main action for attaining this goal, it is not the only thing that needs to be done. Some sub-actions might include diet modifications such as:

- Sustain a balanced healthy diet, predominantly vegetables, fruit, whole grains and low-fat meat and dairy.
- Drink more water.

Although these sub-actions aren't explicitly stated in the goal statement they include other things that you would do in order to imrpove your physical health. They align with the overall goal statement.

On the other hand, the following sub-actions would be misaligned because there is a lack of alignment with accomplishing the goal:

* Not following a healthy, balanced diet

* Not exercising regularly.

Ultimately a person will not be able to maintain their physical wellbeing without completing these sub-actions. This demonstrates that implementing alignment makes it easier to achieve goals.

A student told us …

I set goals but have trouble accomplishing them.

CHECK LIST Checklist to ensure it all aligns

☐ Review your goals and ensure you can track your progress

☐ Make sure the sub-actions are consistent with achieving your overall goals

☐ Review your core values and ensure they align with your purpose

☐ Examine how you are connected to more, or plan to be, and identify how this allows you to fulfil your purpose

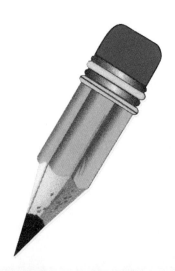

DIY: Does it all align?

Work through the following activities to check your understanding of alignment and ensure that it is present in your life.

1   Are the following statements true or false?

   a   **True or False**   Only focusing on life at the individual level fulfils your purpose.

   b   **True or False**   Practising calmness helps improve your mindset.

   c   **True or False**   You can maintain a healthy mindset by only reacting in situations where someone makes you really upset.

2   Do your health and wellbeing goals align?

   a   Go back to Section 8 and review the goals you wrote in the activity: 'What are your health and wellbeing goals?' (See p. 94)

   b   Add those goals to the table below.

   c   Next, detail some sub-actions for attaining those goals.

   d   Finally, review it all and determine whether it all aligns.

   e   If it doesn't, how can you modify the sub-actions to bring everything into alignment?

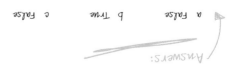

a False   b True   c False

Answers:

Goal:	Is there alignment? (yes/no)
Sub-actions:	

Goal:	Is there alignment? (yes/no)
Sub-actions:	

Goal:	Is there alignment? (yes/no)
Sub-actions:	

Goal:	Is there alignment? (yes/no)
Sub-actions:	

Goal:	Is there alignment? (yes/no)
Sub-actions:	

Goal:	Is there alignment? (yes/no)
Sub-actions:	

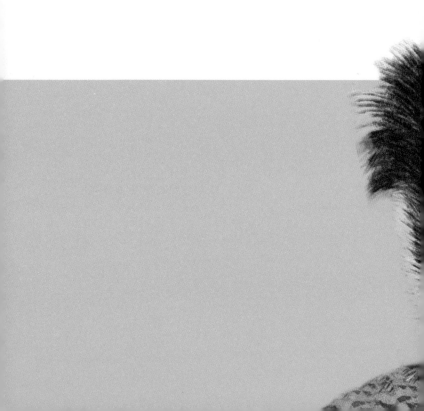

Congratulations

on learning how to ensure everything aligns to help you successfully achieve your goals!

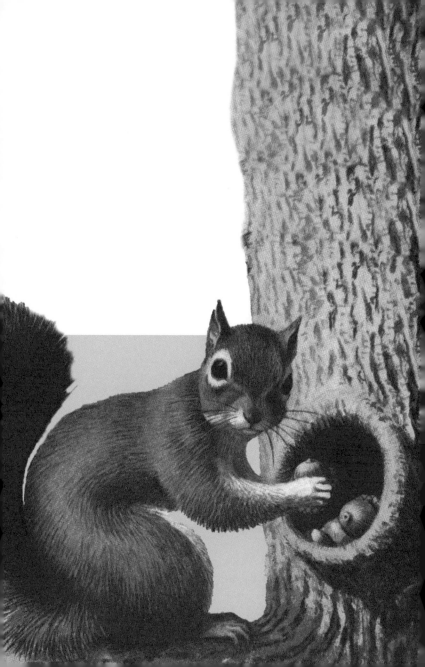

Final checklist:
How to know
you are done

1   I understand what wellbeing comprises   ☐

2   I will make an effort to have a diet of mainly whole
plant-based food sources and to limit processed foods,
meat, dairy, foods high in fat and foods high in sugar   ☐

3   I will do aerobic cardiovascular exercise at least
3 times a week for at least 30 mins   ☐

4   I understand the importance of using proper form
and technique to prevent injuries while resistance training   ☐

5   I have strategies to practise self-awareness and
overcome negative thinking   ☐

6   I have identified the important relationships in my life
    and ways in which they can be improved

7   I have identified my core values and am closer to
    recognizing my purpose in life

8   I can set achievable goals which include an area
    of improvement, time frame and actions

9   I will continually examine my actions to ensure they
    align with my core values and the intentions I have
    to achieve goals in all areas of my life

Glossary

Active listening   Active listening means quieting your thoughts and internal filters. It includes making an effort to hear out the other person and understand their perspective.

Alignment   Alignment means that a set of actions are consistent with accomplishing a greater task or goal.

Cardiovascular exercise   Aerobic exercise that elevates your heart rate above your resting heart rate for a sustained period of time.

Core values   The principles and beliefs that guide your life.

Exercise   Exercise or physical activity includes cardiovascular exercise and resistance training.

High-intensity interval training or HIIT   Training that incorporates intervals of aerobic and anaerobic activity.

Mental wellbeing Mental wellbeing is inclusive of our thoughts, relationships and a connection to something beyond ourselves. Our thoughts, in particular the things we say to ourselves, affect our mental wellbeing.

Mindset The way your think about life, how you view situations and your overall outlook on life.

Nutrition Nutrition includes the nutrients you receive from consuming food.

Physical wellbeing (health) Physical wellbeing relates to the health of the body. Our diet or the food we eat and the amount of exercise we do affects the health of the body.

Purpose How you see your life helping others. You may have a particular talent or skill that you can use to help others.

Resistance training Resistance training includes activities such as lifting weights, using resistance bands or other types of training where the goal is to build muscle.

Rest Rest is another component that contributes to your physical wellbeing and includes refraining from physical activity to allow the body to recover.

Self-awareness This is the ability to observe and self-reflect upon one's own thinking.

Toxic relationships Relationships that lack the components of healthy relationships are discussed in Sections 5 and 6. These are relationships that are harmful to your wellbeing.

Wellbeing Wellbeing refers to the overall health and wellness of an individual. The components of your wellbeing are both physical and mental.

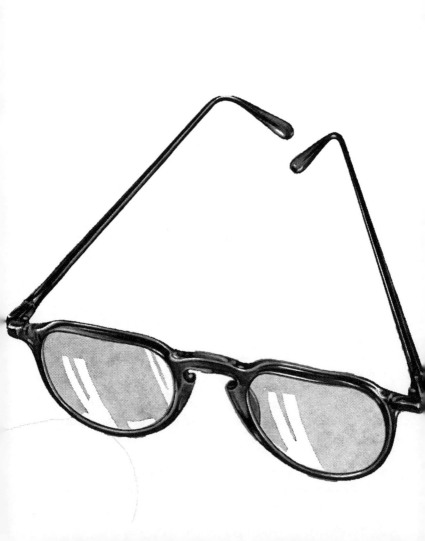

Further reading and resources

Nutrition.gov provides some general resources about healthy eating and nutrition:

www.nutrition.gov

You can learn more about nutrition at Eat Right:

www.eatright.org/food

The NHS website includes a variety of information related to overall health and wellbeing including resources for nutrition, exercise and mental wellbeing:

www.nhs.uk

For more information on how to get started with exercising, ACE Fitness provides a library of exercises and workouts as well as access to certified professional trainers:

www.acefitness.org/education-and-resources/lifestyle/exercise-library

Mind is a mental health charity that provides resources and support for mental health:

www.mind.org.uk